EAT TO LIVE ,NOT TO DIE

HEALTHY NUTRITION

BHANU PRASAD R

Made with ♥ on the Notion Press Platform
www.notionpress.com

KILL THE DISEASE BEFORE IT KILLS YOU .

BY BHANU PRASAD

"

"THIS BOOK I AM DEDICATING TO ALL THE PEOPLE WHO ALL ARE SUFFERING FROM VARIOUS DISEASES "

Contents

Foreword

"EXCERCISE IS THE KING . NUTRITION IS QUEEN. PUT THEM TOGETHER AND YOU'VE GOT A KINGDOM

Jack Lalanne"

FOODS AND NUTRITION are essential for maintaining good health and to prevent disease.although food occupies in first position in the hierarchical needs for man.good nutrition is a function of both economics and education. In our country,the most serious form of nutritional disorders is undernutrition arising from inadequate purchasing power.

This book covers all the important areas which bought to be taken into consideration while promoting good nutrition in health and disease.

It will also be a valuble book for uses of dietetics,nutritionist,public people and students.

Preface

""HEALTH IS THE FOUNDATION OF A HAPPY LIFE
""

I AM VERY HAPPY, To present this book *"Eat to live" not to die"* .. this book is an introduction to foods,nutrition and diet t .This book contains about *healthy nutrition* .TODAY, more than 95% of all chronic disease is caused by food choice,toxic food ingredients, nutritional deficiencies and lack of physical exercise

<u>ABOUT AUTHOR</u>

I AM <u>*BHANU PRASAD .R*</u> born on 13 december 2004 and Author of this book **"eat to live not to die"** ..I Am Ex -student of shree swaminarayan gurukul Banglore and currently i am doing my graduate in Dayananda sagar university .The author embarked on the mission to improve the health through diet and lifestyle changes and it details about what to eat ,what to avoid.

It also covers nutritional value of different types of vegetables,fruits,cereals and etc..

I am very gratefull to all who have Encouraged me while doing this book especially with be support of my parents ,friends and Lectures ...reach me out in{bhanuprasadr183@gmail.com} ,http://linkedin.com/in/bhanu-prasad-r-b0533628a

*******THANK YOU********

Acknowledgements

*NUTRITION ISN'T JUST ABOUT EATING,
ITS ABOUT LEARNING TO LIVE*

I am very thankful to all nutritionist and dietician for their valuable comments and inputs they have gaven .

CHAPTER I

INTRODUCTION

"IF YOU CAN CHANGE YOUR MIND YOU CAN CHANGE YOUR LIFE
WILLIAM JAMES "

INTRODUCTION ABOUT: *"EAT TO LIVE" 'NOT TO DIE"*

The phrase "eat to live, not to die" emphasizes the importance of adopting healthy eating habits for the purpose of maintaining and improving overall health and well-being, rather than merely avoiding death or disease. This perspective encourages people to view food as nourishment and fuel for the body, prioritizing nutritious, balanced meals that support long-term vitality and quality of life. It's a call to make mindful, health-conscious choices about what we consume, rather than simply eating to stave off hunger or prevent immediate health crises.

Health

It is a state of complete physical, mental, and social well-being, and not merely the absence of disease or infirmity. It encompasses various aspects:

1. Physical Health: Involves the proper functioning of the body and its systems. Good physical health is maintained through regular exercise, a balanced diet, adequate rest, and preventive medical care.

2. Mental Health: Refers to cognitive and emotional well-being. It includes the ability to manage stress, maintain relationships, and make sound decisions. Good mental health allows individuals to cope with the normal stresses of life, work productively, and contribute to their community.

3. Social Health: Involves the ability to form satisfying interpersonal relationships with others and to adapt comfortably to different social situations. It includes effective communication skills, empathy, and the ability to develop a support network.

4. Environmental Health: Focuses on the interrelationship between people and their environment. It includes ensuring clean air and water, safe housing, and healthy workplaces.

5. Spiritual Health: Relates to having a sense of purpose and meaning in life, which can be achieved through various means, such as religion, meditation, or a sense of connectedness with the broader universe.

Health is dynamic and can change over time based on lifestyle, environment, genetic factors, and access to healthcare. Maintaining good health involves a holistic approach that balances these different aspects to achieve overall well-being.

<u>"FOOD"</u>

It is any substance consumed to provide nutritional support for the body. It is usually derived from plants, animals, or fungi, and contains essential nutrients, such as carbohydrates, fats, proteins, vitamins, and minerals. These nutrients are crucial for:

1. Energy: Food provides the energy needed for all bodily functions, from basic metabolic processes to physical activities.

2. Growth and Development: Nutrients in food are necessary for the growth and development of tissues, muscles, bones, and organs, especially during childhood and adolescence.

3. Maintenance and Repair: Food helps maintain and repair body tissues, ensuring the proper functioning of organs and systems.

4. Regulation of Body Processes: Vitamins, minerals, and other nutrients play key roles in regulating bodily processes, such as hormone production, immune function, and metabolism.

<u>**Food can be categorized into different groups based on its nutritional composition and origin:**</u>

1. Fruits and Vegetables: Rich in vitamins, minerals, fiber, and antioxidants.

2. Grains and Cereals: Provide carbohydrates, fiber, and essential nutrients.

3. Proteins: Including meat, fish, eggs, legumes, and nuts, which are vital for muscle repair and immune function.

4. Dairy: Sources of calcium, protein, and vitamins.

5. Fats and Oils: Important for energy, cell structure, and hormone production.

Food can be categorized into different groups based on its nutritional composition and origin:

1. Fruits and Vegetables: Rich in vitamins, minerals, fiber, and antioxidants.

2. Grains and Cereals: Provide carbohydrates, fiber, and essential nutrients.

3. Proteins: Including meat, fish, eggs, legumes, and nuts, which are vital for muscle repair and immune function.

4. Dairy: Sources of calcium, protein, and vitamins.

5. Fats and Oils: Important for energy, cell structure, and hormone production.

CHAPTER II

NUTRITION AND DIET

"OUR FOOD SHOULD BE OUR MEDICINE AND OUR MEDICINE SHOULD BE OUR FOOD
HIPPOCRATES "

Nutrition and Diet

They are interrelated concepts that play crucial roles in maintaining health and well-being:

Nutrition

Nutrition refers to the process by which organisms take in and utilize food substances. It involves:

1. Nutrients: Essential substances that the body needs to function correctly. These include:

- **Macronutrients**: Carbohydrates, proteins, and fats, which provide energy and are necessary for growth and repair.

- **Micronutrients**: Vitamins and minerals required in smaller amounts but essential for various bodily functions.

- **Water**: Vital for maintaining hydration, regulating body temperature, and facilitating various biochemical reactions.

2. Functions of Nutrients:

- **Energy Production**: Carbohydrates and fats are the primary sources of energy.

- **Growth and Maintenance**: Proteins are crucial for building and repairing tissues.

- **Regulation of Body Processes**: Vitamins and minerals play key roles in metabolic pathways, immune function, and overall health.

3. Balanced Nutrition: Involves consuming a variety of foods to ensure the body gets all the necessary nutrients in appropriate amounts. This helps prevent deficiencies and supports overall

health.

DIET

Diet refers to the habitual consumption of food and drink by an individual. It encompasses:

1. Dietary Patterns: The types, quantities, and combinations of foods and beverages consumed regularly. Examples include vegetarian, Mediterranean, ketogenic, and traditional diets.

2. Dietary Guidelines: Recommendations provided by health organizations to help individuals make healthy food choices. These guidelines typically emphasize:

- **Variety**: Eating a wide range of foods to ensure a balanced intake of nutrients.

- **Moderation**: Consuming foods and beverages in appropriate portions to maintain a healthy weight and avoid overconsumption of unhealthy foods.

- **Balance**: Ensuring that the intake of calories and nutrients aligns with an individual's energy expenditure and nutritional needs.

3. Special Diets: Specific dietary plans designed to address particular health conditions, dietary restrictions, or lifestyle choices. Examples include gluten-free diets for those with celiac disease, low-carb diets for weight loss, and plant-based diets for ethical or environmental reasons.

RELATIONSHIP BETWEEN NUTRITION AND DIET

- **Quality of Diet**: A diet rich in nutrient-dense foods (such as fruits, vegetables, whole grains, lean proteins, and healthy fats) promotes good nutrition and supports overall health.

- **Nutritional Deficiencies**: Poor dietary habits (such as excessive intake of processed foods, sugars, and unhealthy fats) can lead to nutritional deficiencies and associated health problems.

- **Individual Needs**: Nutritional requirements can vary based on age, gender, health status, and activity level, making it important to tailor diet plans to meet individual needs.

VEGETABLES AND THERE NUTRITIONAL USES

They are a diverse group of plant-based foods that provide a wide range of essential nutrients and health benefits. Including a variety of vegetables in your diet is crucial for overall health. Here are different types of vegetables, their nutritional profiles, and the health benefits they offer:

Leafy Green Vegetables

Examples: Spinach, kale, Swiss chard, arugula, lettuce, collard greens

Nutritional Profile:

- Rich in vitamins A, C, K, and folate

- High in iron, calcium, and magnesium

- Excellent source of fiber and antioxidants

Health Benefits:

- Supports bone health (due to calcium and vitamin K)

- Promotes healthy vision and skin (vitamin A)

- Boosts immune function (vitamin C)

- Reduces inflammation and oxidative stress (antioxidants)

Cruciferous Vegetables

Examples: Broccoli, cauliflower, Brussels sprouts, cabbage, bok choy

Nutritional Profile:

- High in vitamins C, K, and folate

- Contains fiber, potassium, and phytonutrients like glucosinolates

- Low in calories

Health Benefits:

- May reduce the risk of certain cancers (glucosinolates)

- Supports cardiovascular health

- Aids digestion and promotes gut health (fiber)

- Enhances detoxification processes

Root Vegetables

Examples: Carrots, sweet potatoes, beets, radishes, turnips

Nutritional Profile:

- Rich in vitamins A (carotenoids), C, and B6

- Good source of potassium, manganese, and fiber

- Contains natural sugars and complex carbohydrates

Health Benefits:
- Improves vision and immune function (vitamin A)
- Supports cardiovascular health (potassium)
- Aids in digestion and bowel regularity (fiber)
- Provides sustained energy (complex carbohydrates)

Allium Vegetables

Examples: Garlic, onions, leeks, shallots, chives

Nutritional Profile:
- Contains vitamins C and B6, manganese, and selenium
- Rich in sulfur compounds like allicin
- Provides antioxidants and flavonoids

Health Benefits:
- May reduce blood pressure and cholesterol levels
- Supports immune function and fights infections (allicin)
- Enhances detoxification and liver health
- Possesses anti-inflammatory properties

Nightshade Vegetables

Examples: Tomatoes, bell peppers, eggplants, potatoes

Nutritional Profile:
- High in vitamins C, A, and B6
- Contains potassium, folate, and fiber
- Rich in antioxidants like lycopene (tomatoes)

Health Benefits:
- Promotes heart health (potassium and fiber)
- Supports immune function (vitamin C)
- May reduce the risk of certain cancers (lycopene)
- Improves skin health and vision (vitamin A)

Legumes (Podded Vegetables)

Examples: Green beans, peas, lentils, chickpeas, soybeans

Nutritional Profile:
- High in protein, fiber, and complex carbohydrates
- Contains vitamins B1, B6, folate, and minerals like iron and magnesium
- Low in fat and calories

Health Benefits:
- Supports muscle growth and repair (protein)
- Aids in digestion and bowel health (fiber)
- Helps regulate blood sugar levels (complex carbohydrates)
- Reduces the risk of chronic diseases like heart disease and diabetes

Squash and Gourds
Examples: Zucchini, pumpkin, butternut squash, cucumber
Nutritional Profile:
- Rich in vitamins A, C, and B-complex vitamins
- Good source of fiber, potassium, and magnesium
- Contains antioxidants like beta-carotene (pumpkin)

<u>Health Benefits:</u>
- Supports immune function and skin health (vitamin A and C)
- Aids in hydration (high water content in cucumbers)
- Promotes healthy digestion (fiber)
- May help regulate blood pressure (potassium)

<u>BENEFITS OF INCLUDING A VARIETY OF VEGETABLES IN YOUR DIET</u>

- *Nutrient Density:* Vegetables are low in calories but high in vitamins, minerals, and other essential nutrients.

- *Disease Prevention:* Regular consumption of vegetables is linked to a lower risk of chronic diseases such as heart disease, diabetes, and certain cancers.

- *Weight Management:* High fiber content in vegetables can promote satiety and help with weight management.

- *Digestive Health*: Fiber in vegetables supports healthy digestion and prevents constipation.

- *Antioxidant Protection*: Antioxidants in vegetables help protect the body from oxidative stress and inflammation.

<u>FRUITS AND THERE NUTRITIONAL USES ARE</u>

''A vital part of a healthy diet due to their high nutrient content and numerous health benefits. Different fruits provide various vitamins, minerals, antioxidants, and dietary fiber, all of which contribute to overall health and can help prevent or manage certain diseases. Here's a look at some common fruits and their nutritional profiles, health benefits, and potential roles in disease prevention"

Common Fruits and Their Nutritional Profiles

1. Apples

- Nutritional Content: Rich in dietary fiber, vitamin C, and various antioxidants.

- Health Benefits: May reduce the risk of heart disease, promote gut health, and help with weight management.

- Disease Prevention: The antioxidants in apples may help lower the risk of chronic diseases such as heart disease and cancer.

2. Bananas

- Nutritional Content: High in potassium, vitamin C, vitamin B6, and fiber.

- Health Benefits: Good for heart health, digestive health, and energy production.

- Disease Prevention: Potassium helps regulate blood pressure, reducing the risk of hypertension and stroke.

3. Berries (Strawberries, Blueberries, Raspberries)

- Nutritional Content: Packed with vitamins (C and K), fiber, and antioxidants like anthocyanins.

- Health Benefits: Improve heart health, cognitive function, and blood sugar regulation.

- Disease Prevention: High antioxidant content helps reduce inflammation and oxidative stress, lowering the risk of chronic diseases such as cancer and heart disease.

4. Citrus Fruits (Oranges, Lemons, Grapefruits

- Nutritional Content: High in vitamin C, fiber, and various antioxidants.

- Health Benefits: Boost immune function, improve skin health, and support cardiovascular health.

- Disease Prevention: Vitamin C and flavonoids in citrus fruits can help reduce inflammation and the risk of chronic diseases like heart disease and cancer.

5. Grapes

- Nutritional Content: Contain vitamins C and K, antioxidants (resveratrol), and fiber.

- Health Benefits: Support heart health, improve blood sugar control, and enhance brain function.

- Disease Prevention: Resveratrol and other antioxidants may help reduce the risk of heart disease, cancer, and neurodegenerative diseases.

6. **Pineapples**

- Nutritional Content: High in vitamin C, manganese, and bromelain (an enzyme).

- Health Benefits: Aids digestion, reduces inflammation, and supports immune function.

- Disease Prevention: Bromelain has anti-inflammatory properties and may help reduce the risk of certain cancers.

7. **Mangoes**

- Nutritional Content: Rich in vitamins A and C, fiber, and antioxidants.

- Health Benefits: Promote eye health, boost immune function, and improve digestion.

- Disease Prevention: High levels of antioxidants and vitamins can help reduce the risk of chronic diseases like cancer and heart disease.

8. **Avocados**

- Nutritional Content: High in healthy fats (monounsaturated fats), fiber, vitamins E, C, B6, and potassium.

- Health Benefits: Support heart health, improve digestion, and provide anti-inflammatory benefits.

- Disease Prevention: The healthy fats and antioxidants in avocados may help lower the risk of heart disease and improve overall health.

Specific Health Benefits and Disease Prevention

- ***Heart Health:*** Fruits rich in fiber, potassium, and antioxidants, such as bananas, berries, and citrus fruits, can help lower blood pressure, reduce cholesterol levels, and decrease the risk of heart disease.

- _**Digestive Health:**_ High-fiber fruits like apples, pears, and berries promote healthy digestion and prevent constipation.

- _**Immune Function:**_ Vitamin C-rich fruits like citrus fruits, strawberries, and kiwis boost immune function and help protect against infections.

- **Cancer Prevention**: Antioxidant-rich fruits like berries, grapes, and citrus fruits help neutralize free radicals and reduce the risk of cancer.

- _**Anti-Inflammatory Benefits:**_ Fruits like pineapples (bromelain), berries, and avocados have anti-inflammatory properties that can help manage conditions like arthritis and reduce overall inflammation.

DIETARY RECOMMENDATIONS

Incorporating a variety of fruits into your daily diet can provide a wide range of nutrients and health benefits. Aim for at least 2-3 servings of fruit per day, choosing different colors and types to ensure a diverse intake of vitamins, minerals, and antioxidants. Fresh, frozen, and canned fruits (without added sugars) are all good options.

By maintaining a balanced diet that includes a variety of fruits, you can support overall health, prevent nutrient deficiencies, and reduce the risk of many chronic diseases.

**TYPES OF CEREALS AND THERE NUTRITIONAL USES**

Oats

Nutritional Benefits:

- **High in Fiber**: Particularly soluble fiber (beta-glucan), which can help lower cholesterol levels.
- **Rich in Vitamins and Minerals**: Includes manganese, phosphorus, magnesium, copper, iron, zinc, folate, and vitamins B1 and B5.
- **Contains Antioxidants**: Including avenanthramides, which can help reduce blood pressure.

Health and Diet:

- **Heart Health**: The fiber in oats can help reduce LDL cholesterol levels.
- **Weight Management**: Oats can promote satiety and reduce overall calorie intake.
- **Digestive Health**: High fiber content aids in digestion and prevents constipation.

Disease Prevention:

- **Cardiovascular Disease**: Regular consumption can lower the risk of heart disease.
- **Type 2 Diabetes**: The fiber in oats can help control blood sugar levels.

2. Quinoa
Nutritional Benefits:

- **Complete Protein**: Contains all nine essential amino acids.
- **High in Fiber**: More fiber than most other grains.
- **Rich in Vitamins and Minerals**: Includes magnesium, iron, potassium, and calcium.
- **Gluten-Free**: Suitable for those with gluten intolerance or celiac disease.

Health and Diet:

- **Muscle Health**: The complete protein content supports muscle repair and growth.
- **Digestive Health**: High fiber content aids digestion.
- **Bone Health**: Contains calcium and magnesium, which are essential for bone health.

Disease Prevention:

- **Inflammation**: Contains anti-inflammatory phytonutrients.

- **Heart Disease**: Fiber and antioxidants can reduce the risk of cardiovascular disease.
- **Cancer**: Potential anti-cancer properties due to its nutrient and antioxidant content.

3. Brown Rice
Nutritional Benefits:

- **High in Fiber**: Helps with digestion and maintaining a healthy weight.
- **Rich in Selenium and Manganese**: Essential for immune function and antioxidant defense.
- **Contains Magnesium**: Important for numerous biochemical reactions in the body.

Health and Diet:

- **Blood Sugar Control**: Lower glycemic index compared to white rice, which helps control blood sugar levels.
- **Weight Management**: High fiber content promotes satiety.
- **Digestive Health**: Fiber aids in regular bowel movements.

Disease Prevention:

- **Type 2 Diabetes**: Can help lower the risk of developing diabetes.
- **Heart Disease**: Fiber, selenium, and magnesium contribute to heart health.
- **Cancer**: The selenium content may help reduce the risk of certain cancers.

4. Barley
Nutritional Benefits:

- **High in Fiber**: Especially beta-glucans, which can help lower cholesterol.

- **Rich in Vitamins and Minerals**: Includes selenium, B vitamins, and manganese.
- **Contains Antioxidants**: Such as lignans, which can provide health benefits.

Health and Diet:

- **Heart Health**: The beta-glucan fiber can help reduce cholesterol and improve heart health.
- **Weight Management**: Fiber promotes satiety and reduces overall calorie intake.
- **Digestive Health**: High fiber content helps with regular bowel movements and digestive health.

Disease Prevention:

- **Cardiovascular Disease**: Can help lower cholesterol and improve heart health.
- **Type 2 Diabetes**: Fiber helps control blood sugar levels.
- **Cancer**: Antioxidants and fiber may reduce the risk of certain cancers.

5. Millet
Nutritional Benefits:

- **High in Fiber**: Helps with digestion and weight management.
- **Rich in Magnesium**: Important for heart health and metabolic functions.
- **Contains Antioxidants**: Such as phenolic acids and flavonoids.

Health and Diet:

- **Blood Sugar Control**: Low glycemic index, which helps control blood sugar levels.

- **Digestive Health**: Fiber aids in digestion and prevents constipation.
- **Bone Health**: Contains magnesium, which is important for bone health.

Disease Prevention:

- **Heart Disease**: Magnesium and fiber contribute to heart health.
- **Type 2 Diabetes**: Helps control blood sugar levels.
- **Inflammation**: Antioxidants help reduce inflammation in the body.

<u>MEAT: NUTRITIONAL HEALTH, DIET, AND DISEASE</u>

Nutritional Health: Meat is a rich source of essential nutrients that play vital roles in the body's overall health:

1. **Proteins**: High-quality proteins are essential for muscle repair, growth, and maintenance. Meat provides all the essential amino acids needed by the body.
2. **Vitamins:**

   - **B Vitamins**: Particularly B12, which is crucial for nerve function and blood cell production. B6 helps with brain development and function.
   - **Vitamin D**: Found in fatty fish and liver, it is important for bone health and immune function.

3. **Minerals:**

   - **Iron**: Especially heme iron, which is more readily absorbed by the body. Iron is vital for oxygen transport in the blood.
   - **Zinc**: Important for immune function, wound healing, and DNA synthesis.
   - **Selenium**: Acts as an antioxidant, protecting cells from damage.

Meat in Diet:

1. **Types of Meat:**

   - **Red Meat:** Beef, lamb, and pork. Rich in iron and B vitamins but should be consumed in moderation.
   - **White Meat:** Chicken and turkey. Lower in fat compared to red meat and a good source of lean protein.
   - **Fish and Seafood:** High in omega-3 fatty acids, which are beneficial for heart health.

2. **Moderation and Balance:**

   - Incorporate a variety of protein sources, including plant-based options, to ensure a balanced diet.
   - Opt for lean cuts and avoid processed meats to reduce the intake of unhealthy fats and additives.

3. **Healthy Preparation:**

   - Grilling, baking, or steaming instead of frying.
   - Removing visible fat and skin to reduce saturated fat intake.

Meat and Disease:

1. **Positive Health Impacts:**

   - **Anemia Prevention:** Iron-rich meats help prevent iron-deficiency anemia.
   - **Muscle Health:** High-quality protein supports muscle mass and function, important for aging populations.
   - **Brain Function:** B12 and omega-3 fatty acids found in meat are crucial for cognitive health.

2. **Potential Risks:**

- **Heart Disease**: High consumption of red and processed meats has been linked to an increased risk of heart disease due to high saturated fat and cholesterol content.
- **Cancer**: Some studies suggest a link between high intake of processed and red meats and an increased risk of certain cancers, particularly colorectal cancer.
- **Inflammation**: Excessive meat consumption, especially processed meats, may contribute to inflammation and related chronic diseases.

Meat and Disease Prevention:

1. **Balanced Diet**:

   - Combining meat with plenty of fruits, vegetables, whole grains, and legumes can help offset potential negative health effects.
   - Focusing on lean meats and healthier cooking methods can reduce the risk of disease.

2. **Specific Diets for Health Conditions**:

   - **Mediterranean Diet**: Emphasizes lean meats like fish and poultry, alongside plant-based foods, and has been associated with lower risks of heart disease and cancer.
   - **DASH Diet (Dietary Approaches to Stop Hypertension)**: Recommends moderate meat intake with an emphasis on lean proteins, which can help manage blood pressure.

3. **Role in Healing and Recovery**:

   - **Post-Surgery Recovery**: High-protein diets can support tissue repair and recovery after surgery.
   - **Elderly Nutrition**: Ensuring adequate protein intake helps maintain muscle mass and strength, reducing the risk of falls

and fractures.

CHAPTER III

LIFESTYLE MODIFICATION OF CARDIAC

Lifestyle modifications, especially in terms of nutrition and diet, play a crucial role in managing heart disease. Here are some recommendations for cardiac patients:

1. Adopt a Heart-Healthy Diet:

A. Increase Intake of Fruits and Vegetables:

Aim for at least 5 servings of fruits and vegetables per day.

Include a variety of colors to ensure a wide range of nutrients.

B. Choose Whole Grains:

Opt for whole grain bread, brown rice, oats, and whole wheat pasta.

Whole grains are rich in fiber, which can help lower cholesterol levels.

C. Healthy Protein Sources:

Prefer lean meats like chicken or turkey without the skin.

Incorporate fish, especially fatty fish like salmon, mackerel, and sardines, which are high in omega-3 fatty acids.

Include plant-based proteins like beans, lentils, tofu, and nuts.

2. Limit Unhealthy Fats:

Reduce saturated fats found in red meat, butter, cheese, and full-fat dairy products.

Avoid trans fats found in many processed foods, margarine, and commercially baked products.

Use healthier fats like olive oil, canola oil, and avocados.

3. Reduce Sodium Intake:

Limit sodium to less than 2,300 milligrams per day, or even less if advised by your doctor.

Avoid adding extra salt to your meals.

Check food labels and choose low-sodium options.

Limit intake of processed and restaurant foods, which are often high in salt.

4. Increase Fiber Intake:

Consume soluble fiber, which can help lower cholesterol. Foods rich in soluble fiber include oats, barley, beans, and fruits.

Aim for 25-30 grams of fiber per day.

5. Control Portion Sizes:

Be mindful of portion sizes to avoid overeating.

Use smaller plates and bowls to help control portions.

Read food labels to understand serving sizes.

6. Stay Hydrated:

Drink plenty of water throughout the day.

Limit sugary drinks and excessive caffeine.

7. Limit Alcohol:

If you drink alcohol, do so in moderation. This generally means up to one drink per day for women and up to two drinks per day for men.

8. Plan Balanced Meals:

Aim for balanced meals that include a combination of protein, carbohydrates, and healthy fats.

Include a variety of food groups to ensure adequate nutrient intake.

9. Read Food Labels:

Pay attention to food labels to make healthier choices.

Look for foods low in saturated fat, trans fat, cholesterol, and sodium

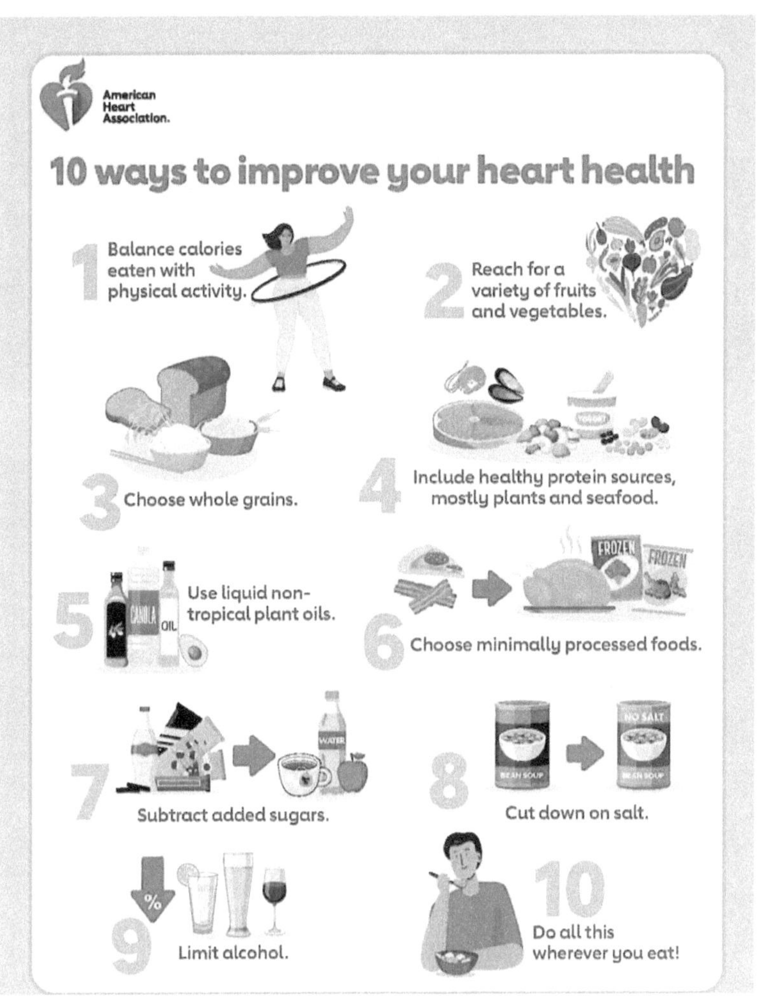

Enter Caption

CANCER

Lifestyle modifications, particularly in nutrition and diet, play a crucial role in supporting cancer patients during treatment and recovery. Here are some key considerations:

General Principles

Balanced Diet: Ensure a diet that includes a variety of foods to provide essential nutrients.

High Protein: Protein helps repair body tissue and maintain immune function. Include lean meats, poultry, fish, eggs, dairy, beans, nuts, and soy products.

High Calorie: Some patients may need more calories to maintain their weight during treatment.

Hydration: Adequate fluid intake is essential to prevent dehydration.

Small, Frequent Meals: Eating smaller, more frequent meals can help manage appetite loss and nausea.

Specific Recommendations

Fruits and Vegetables: Aim for a variety of colorful fruits and vegetables. They provide essential vitamins, minerals, and antioxidants.

Whole Grains: Include whole grains like brown rice, whole wheat bread, oatmeal, and quinoa.

Healthy Fats: Opt for sources of healthy fats such as avocados, nuts, seeds, and olive oil.

Limit Processed Foods: Reduce intake of processed foods, sugary snacks, and red meats.

Limit Alcohol: Alcohol consumption should be minimized or avoided.

Avoid Food Safety Risks: Be cautious with raw or undercooked foods to prevent foodborne illnesses.

Managing Treatment Side Effects

Nausea and Vomiting: Ginger tea, peppermint, small meals, and bland foods can help manage nausea.

Loss of Appetite: High-calorie snacks, meal replacements, and nutrient-dense foods can help maintain energy levels.

Mouth Sores: Soft, non-acidic foods, and avoiding spicy or acidic foods can help reduce discomfort.

Diarrhea: Hydration, electrolytes, and avoiding high-fiber foods can help manage diarrhea.

Constipation: Increase fiber intake and fluid consumption, and consider light physical activity.

Supplements

Vitamins and Minerals: Some patients may require supplements to address deficiencies. Consult a healthcare provider before starting any supplements.

Omega-3 Fatty Acids: Found in fish oil, these can help with inflammation and overall health.

Consultation

Registered Dietitian: Working with a dietitian specialized in oncology can provide personalized nutrition plans.

Oncologist: Always consult with the treating oncologist before making significant dietary changes or adding supplements.

Emotional and Psychological Support

Support Groups: Emotional well-being is crucial. Support groups and counseling can help manage stress and emotional challenges.

CHOLESTEROL

Modifying lifestyle, particularly nutrition and diet, can significantly impact cholesterol levels. Here are some dietary and lifestyle changes that can help manage cholesterol:

Dietary Modifications:

Increase Soluble Fiber Intake:

Foods high in soluble fiber help reduce the absorption of cholesterol into your bloodstream.

Examples: Oats, barley, beans, lentils, fruits (apples, pears, prunes), and vegetables (carrots, Brussels sprouts).

Choose Healthy Fats:

Replace saturated fats with monounsaturated and polyunsaturated fats.

Sources of healthy fats: Olive oil, canola oil, avocados, nuts, and fatty fish (salmon, mackerel).

Reduce Saturated and Trans Fats:

Limit foods high in saturated fats such as red meat, butter, cheese, and other full-fat dairy products.

Avoid trans fats found in many processed and fried foods.

Increase Omega-3 Fatty Acids:

Omega-3s help lower triglycerides, another type of fat in your blood.

Sources: Fatty fish (salmon, mackerel, sardines), flaxseeds, chia seeds, and walnuts.

Add Plant Sterols and Stanols:

These substances, found in plants, help block the absorption of cholesterol.

Foods fortified with sterols and stanols include some margarine, orange juice, and yogurt drinks.

Limit Dietary Cholesterol:

Found in animal products like egg yolks, shrimp, and organ meats.

Aim for less than 200 mg of cholesterol per day if you are at risk of high cholesterol.

Eat a Variety of Fruits and Vegetables:

These foods are rich in dietary fiber, vitamins, and minerals which can help lower cholesterol levels.

Reduce Sodium Intake:

High sodium can raise blood pressure, which is a risk factor for heart disease.

Limit processed and packaged foods and choose low-sodium options.

Lifestyle Modifications:

Maintain a Healthy Weight:

Losing even a small amount of weight can help lower cholesterol levels.

Exercise Regularly:

Aim for at least 30 minutes of moderate to vigorous exercise most days of the week.

Activities: Walking, jogging, swimming, cycling.

Quit Smoking:

Smoking lowers HDL (good cholesterol) and increases the risk of heart disease.

Limit Alcohol Consumption:

Moderate alcohol consumption can have heart benefits, but too much can increase cholesterol and triglycerides.

Guidelines: Up to one drink per day for women and two drinks per day for men.

Manage Stress:

Chronic stress may contribute to higher cholesterol levels.

Techniques: Meditation, yoga, deep breathing exercises, and other relaxation techniques.

DIABETES MELLITUS

Lifestyle modifications, particularly in nutrition and diet, are crucial for managing diabetes effectively. Here are some key strategies:

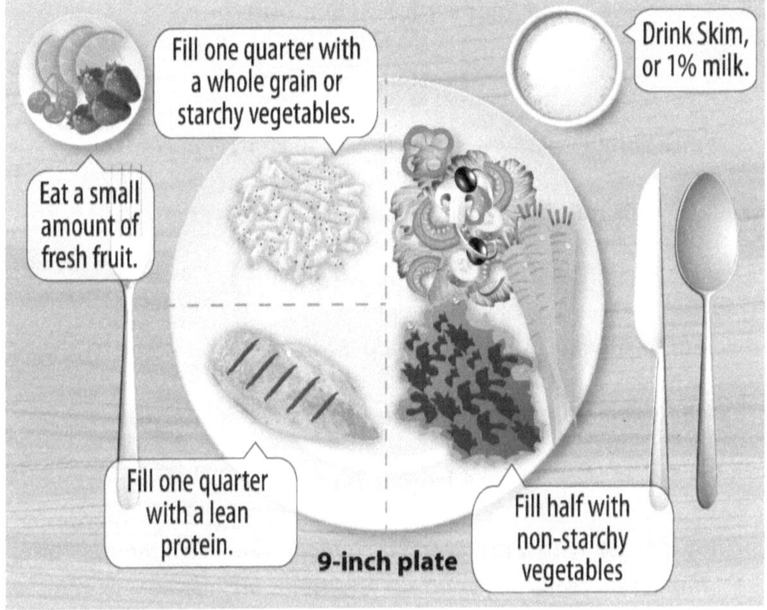

Enter Caption

Nutrition and Diet

Balanced Diet:

Carbohydrates: Choose complex carbs like whole grains, vegetables, fruits, and legumes over simple carbs like sugar and refined grains.

Protein: Include lean protein sources such as poultry, fish, beans, and low-fat dairy.

Fats: Opt for healthy fats from nuts, seeds, avocados, and olive oil, and limit saturated and trans fats.

Portion Control:

Use smaller plates and bowls to help control portion sizes.

Be mindful of serving sizes to avoid overeating.

Regular Meals:

Eat at regular intervals to help maintain blood sugar levels.

Avoid skipping meals to prevent blood sugar spikes and crashes.

Low Glycemic Index Foods:

Choose foods with a low glycemic index (GI), which have a slower impact on blood sugar levels. Examples include non-starchy vegetables, most fruits, and whole grains.

Fiber-Rich Foods:

Include plenty of fiber-rich foods such as vegetables, fruits, legumes, and whole grains. Fiber helps slow down the absorption of sugar.

Limit Sugar and Refined Carbs:

Reduce the intake of sugary drinks, candies, pastries, and other sweets.

Replace sugary snacks with healthier options like nuts, seeds, or a piece of fruit.

Healthy Snacking:

Opt for healthy snacks like fresh fruit, raw vegetables, yogurt, or a handful of nuts to keep blood sugar levels stable.

Hydration:

Drink plenty of water throughout the day. Avoid sugary drinks and limit fruit juices.

Moderation with Alcohol:

If you drink alcohol, do so in moderation and always with food to prevent blood sugar fluctuations.

Reading Food Labels:

Learn to read and understand food labels to make healthier choices.

Additional Lifestyle Modifications

Regular Physical Activity:

Aim for at least 150 minutes of moderate-intensity aerobic activity per week, such as brisk walking or cycling.

Include strength training exercises at least twice a week.

Weight Management:

Maintain a healthy weight to help control blood sugar levels. Even a modest weight loss can significantly impact blood sugar control.

Stress Management:

Practice stress-reducing techniques such as yoga, meditation, deep breathing exercises, or hobbies that help you relax.

Regular Monitoring:

Monitor blood sugar levels regularly as advised by your healthcare provider to track how your diet and lifestyle affect your diabetes.

Education and Support:

Seek education about diabetes management from healthcare professionals.

Consider joining a diabetes support group to share experiences and gain support from others.

Benefits

PRACTICAL TIPS FOR INCLUDING MORE FRUITS AND VEGETABLES IN YOUR DIET

1. **Add Fruits to Breakfast:**

   - Include fruits like berries, bananas, or apples in your morning cereal, yogurt, or smoothies.

2. **Snack on Vegetables:**

   - Keep cut vegetables like carrots, celery, and bell peppers handy for quick, healthy snacks.

3. **Incorporate into Meals:**

   - Add vegetables to soups, stews, casseroles, and stir-fries. Use fruits in salads or as a natural dessert option.

4. **Experiment with New Recipes:**

   - Try new recipes that feature fruits and vegetables as main ingredients to keep your diet interesting and varied.

BENEFITS OF A DIET RICH IN FRUITS AND VEGETABLES

1. **Chronic Disease Prevention:**

   - Regular consumption of fruits and vegetables has been linked to a lower risk of chronic diseases, including cardiovascular disease, hypertension, type 2 diabetes, and certain cancers.

2. **Improved Digestive Health:**

- The fiber content in fruits and vegetables promotes healthy digestion and regular bowel movements, reducing the risk of constipation and other digestive disorders.

3. **Enhanced Immune Function:**

- The vitamins, minerals, and antioxidants in fruits and vegetables support a healthy immune system, helping the body fight off infections and illnesses.

4. **Better Weight Management:**

- High-fiber, low-calorie fruits and vegetables can help create a feeling of fullness, reducing overall calorie intake and supporting weight loss or maintenance.

5. **Boosted Mental Health:**

- Some studies suggest that a diet high in fruits and vegetables can positively affect mental health, reducing the risk of depression and anxiety.

<u>The conclusion</u>

In conclusion, nutrition is fundamental to overall health and well-being. It involves understanding how essential nutrients—carbohydrates, proteins, fats, vitamins, minerals, and water—support various bodily functions and contribute to maintaining energy levels, growth, and repair.

A well-balanced diet, which incorporates a variety of nutrient-dense foods, ensures that the body receives all the necessary elements to function optimally. It helps prevent deficiencies, supports immune function, and reduces the risk of chronic diseases.

Good nutritional practices also involve moderation and balance, adapting dietary choices to individual needs and lifestyle factors. By prioritizing nutritious foods and making mindful dietary choices, individuals can enhance their health, manage weight, and improve their quality of life.

THANK YOU